PILATES FOR A BETTER 60+

A Guide to Safe and Effective Exercise for Seniors

Dr. Laurie Miles

Other Books by The Author:

- Chair Yoga for Seniors Over 50: A Comprehensive Guide to Improving Health and Mobility for Active Aging

INTRODUCTION

Pilates is a form of low-impact exercise that has been around for more than a century. It is a gentle yet effective form of exercise that is suitable for people of all ages, including seniors over 60. The focus on controlled movements, balanced alignment, and core stability makes Pilates a great choice for seniors who want to improve their overall health and well-being.

This book is designed specifically for seniors over 60 who are interested in starting Pilates or are looking for a low-impact exercise that can help them maintain their independence, strength, and mobility as they age. Whether you are a beginner or have experience with Pilates, this book provides valuable information and guidance to help you get the most out of your Pilates practice.

In this book, you will learn about the many benefits of Pilates for seniors, including improved balance, enhanced flexibility, increased strength, and reduced risk of falls and other age-related conditions. You will also learn about the different types of Pilates and how to get started with Pilates for seniors, including guidelines for safe exercise, proper form, and proper alignment.

This book includes a comprehensive table of contents that covers everything from the basics of Pilates to more advanced Pilates routines. Whether you are looking for a simple Pilates routine to do at home or you are interested in taking a Pilates class, this book has something for everyone. So let's get started and discover how Pilates can help you stay healthy, active, and independent as you age.

Chapter 1

Introductory to Pilates

<u>What Is Pilates</u>

Pilates is a form of exercise that was invented by Joseph Pilates in the early 20th century. It is a system of movements that focus on strengthening the core muscles, improving posture, and increasing flexibility. Pilates involves a series of controlled, low-impact movements that are performed on a mat or with the use of specialized equipment. These movements are designed to engage the deep muscles of the body, including the abdomen, lower back, and hips. Pilates is a holistic form of exercise that aims to improve not only physical health but also mental and emotional well-being.

Pilates was originally developed as a rehabilitation exercise for wounded soldiers during World War I. Joseph Pilates was a nurse and physical trainer who was working with bedridden soldiers in a hospital. He noticed that many of them suffered from muscle weakness and poor posture due to their prolonged inactivity. He created a system of movements that would target these areas, and eventually called it "Contrology". The term Pilates was later adopted, and the practice has since become widely popular around the world.

Pilates is often referred to as a mind-body exercise because it requires a high level of concentration and focus. Participants must pay attention to their breathing, posture, and movements in order to get the most out of the exercise. This focus on the mind-body connection is what sets Pilates apart from other forms of exercise.

Pilates is also known for its low-impact nature, making it an ideal form of exercise for people of all ages, including seniors over 60. It is a safe and effective way for older adults to improve their physical health, increase their strength and flexibility, and reduce their risk of injury.

In conclusion, Pilates is a system of movements that was invented to improve physical health, increase strength and flexibility, and promote mental and emotional well-being. It is a mind-body exercise that is low-impact and safe for seniors over 60, making it an ideal form of exercise for older adults.

Benefits of Pilates for Seniors Over 60

Pilates is a great form of exercise for seniors over 60, as it offers a wide range of benefits that are specifically tailored to their needs. Here are some of the top benefits of Pilates for seniors over 60:

- **Improves Balance:**

Pilates movements focus on strengthening the core muscles, which helps improve balance. This is particularly important for seniors, who are more prone to falls.

- **Increases Strength:**

Pilates movements engage the deep muscles of the body, which can help increase strength, especially in the legs, hips, and back.

- **Improves Flexibility:**

Pilates movements are designed to increase flexibility and range of motion. This is especially beneficial for seniors, who may have stiff joints due to arthritis or other conditions.

- **Reduces Pain:**

Pilates can help relieve pain in the lower back, hips, and knees by strengthening the muscles that support these areas.

- **Boosts Mood:**

The mind-body connection in Pilates can help boost mood and reduce stress. This is especially important for seniors, who may be dealing with emotional and mental health issues.

- **Increases Endurance:**

Pilates movements are low-impact, which means they are less likely to cause injury or strain. As a result, seniors can exercise for longer periods of time, increasing their endurance.

In conclusion, Pilates offers a wide range of benefits for seniors over 60, including improved balance, increased strength, improved flexibility, reduced pain, boosted mood, and increased endurance.

<u>Understanding Pilates Movements</u>

Pilates movements are a series of controlled, low-impact exercises that are performed on a mat or with the use of specialized equipment. They focus on strengthening the core muscles, improving posture, and increasing flexibility. There are several different types of Pilates movements, including:

- **Mat exercises:**

These are performed on a mat and involve a series of movements designed to target the core muscles.

- **Equipment-based exercises:**

These are performed with the use of specialized equipment, such as a reformer, Cadillac, or chair.

- **Breathing** exercises:

Pilates places a strong emphasis on proper breathing, which is an important part of the exercise.

Pilates movements are performed in a slow and controlled manner, with a focus on form and alignment. It is important to understand the proper technique for each movement in order to get the most out of the exercise and avoid injury.

Adapting Pilates for Seniors

Pilates can be adapted for seniors in several ways, including:

- **Modifying movements:**

Certain Pilates movements can be modified to make them easier or more challenging, depending on the individual's abilities.

- **Using props:**

Props, such as blocks or straps, can be used to make Pilates movements easier or more challenging.

- **Incorporating modifications for specific conditions:**

Pilates can be adapted for seniors who have specific conditions, such as arthritis, by incorporating modifications that target those areas.

- **Incorporating low-impact movements:**

Pilates movements can be performed in a low-impact manner, making them easier on the joints.

In conclusion, Pilates can be adapted for seniors in several ways, including modifying movements, using props, incorporating modifications for specific conditions, and incorporating low-impact movements. This makes Pilates an accessible and effective form of exercise for seniors over 60.

The Different Types of Pilates

There are several different forms of Pilates that have evolved over the years, each with its own unique set of movements, equipment, and styles. The most common types of Pilates are:

- **Mat Pilates:**

This is the most traditional form of Pilates and involves using a mat and your own body weight for resistance. There is no equipment involved, making it accessible for people of all ages and fitness levels.

- **Reformer Pilates:**

This type of Pilates involves using a machine called a reformer, which provides resistance and stability for the body. This type of Pilates is great for seniors because it helps to improve strength, balance, and stability.

- **Chair Pilates:**

This type of Pilates involves using a chair as a prop to help with balance and stability. It's a great option for seniors who may struggle with getting up and down from the floor.

- **Barrel Pilates:**

This type of Pilates involves using a barrel-shaped piece of equipment to help with strengthening and stretching the spine, hips, and legs.

Chapter 2

Introduction to the Benefits of Pilates for Seniors

Pilates is a low-impact form of exercise that is suitable for people of all ages, including seniors over 60. It provides a range of physical and mental benefits, making it a popular choice for aging individuals who want to maintain their health and wellbeing. In this chapter, we will explore some of the key benefits of Pilates for seniors, including improved flexibility, balance, and strength.

Improved Flexibility

One of the primary benefits of Pilates for seniors is improved flexibility. As we age, our muscles and joints tend to become stiff, leading to a decrease in range of motion and an increased risk of injury. Pilates is designed to help improve flexibility by stretching and lengthening the muscles, increasing the range of motion in the joints, and reducing the risk of injury. Through a series of controlled movements, Pilates helps to improve flexibility in a safe and effective manner, reducing the risk of falls and other accidents.

Enhanced Balance

Another important benefit of Pilates for seniors is enhanced balance. As we age, our balance can deteriorate, leading to an increased risk of falls and other accidents. Pilates helps to improve balance by strengthening the core muscles and improving coordination, allowing seniors to maintain stability and control over their movements. The focus on proper form and alignment in Pilates also helps to improve balance, making it easier for seniors to perform everyday activities and reduce the risk of falls.

Increased Strength

In addition to improving flexibility and balance, Pilates also provides a range of benefits in terms of increased strength. By targeting specific muscle groups, Pilates helps to improve overall strength and endurance, allowing seniors to maintain their independence and perform daily tasks with ease. The low-impact nature of Pilates also makes it a safe and effective form of exercise for seniors, reducing the risk of injury and allowing them to build strength without putting undue stress on their joints.

Improved Mental Health

Finally, Pilates also offers a range of mental health benefits for seniors. The focus on controlled movements and deep breathing can help to reduce stress and anxiety, promoting feelings of calm and relaxation. Pilates also provides an opportunity for seniors to engage in physical activity and socialize with others, promoting a sense of community and helping to combat feelings of isolation and loneliness.

Reduced Risk of Falls and Other Age-Related Conditions: As seniors age, their risk of falls and other age-related conditions like osteoporosis and arthritis increases. Pilates is a low-impact exercise that can help seniors reduce the risk of falls and improve their overall physical health. Through Pilates, seniors can improve their balance, coordination, and overall strength, which in turn helps to reduce the risk of falls. Additionally, Pilates can help to improve flexibility, which can reduce the risk of injury.

Improved Mobility

As seniors age, they can experience a decline in their mobility. This can be due to various factors like arthritis, back pain, and other age-related conditions. Pilates can help seniors to improve their mobility by strengthening their muscles and improving their overall flexibility. Pilates focuses on controlled movements that can help seniors to build strength and improve their range of motion. This, in turn, can help seniors to stay active and move around more easily.

Better Posture

Poor posture is a common problem among seniors, which can lead to a range of issues like back pain and neck pain.

Pilates is designed to improve posture by strengthening the muscles that support the spine. Through Pilates, seniors can learn to engage their core muscles and improve their overall alignment, which can lead to better posture. This can help seniors to reduce the risk of pain and improve their overall comfort.

In conclusion, Pilates provides a range of physical and mental benefits for seniors over 60, including improved flexibility, balance, strength, and mental health. By incorporating Pilates into their routine, seniors can maintain their independence, improve their quality of life, and reduce the risk of injury and accidents.

Chapter 3
Safe Exercise for Seniors

<u>Understanding Age-Related Changes in the Body</u>

As people age, their bodies go through a series of changes that can affect their ability to exercise safely and effectively. Some of these changes include reduced flexibility, decreased muscle mass, and changes in bone density. It's important for seniors to understand these changes and how they can impact their ability to perform physical activities.

One of the most common age-related changes is a decrease in flexibility. As we age, our joints become stiffer, making it more difficult to move freely. This can increase the risk of injury and make it more challenging to perform certain exercises.

Another age-related change is a decrease in muscle mass. Seniors tend to lose muscle mass as they age, which can reduce their strength and endurance. This can make it more difficult to perform physical activities and put them at greater risk of falls.

Finally, changes in bone density can also affect a senior's ability to exercise. As we age, our bones become less dense, making them more fragile and susceptible to fractures. It's important for seniors to be aware of these changes and to take steps to protect their bones while they exercise.

Warm-Up Exercises

Warming up before exercising is important for everyone, but it's especially crucial for seniors. A good warm-up can help increase blood flow, loosen tight muscles, and reduce the risk of injury. Some simple warm-up exercises that seniors can do include:

- **Gentle stretching:**

Stretching can help improve flexibility and prepare the muscles for exercise.

- **Walking:**

A brisk walk can help increase heart rate and get blood flowing to the muscles.

- **Arm swings:**

Swinging the arms can help warm up the shoulders and prepare them for upper body exercises.

It's important for seniors to take their time and listen to their bodies when warming up. If they feel any pain or discomfort, they should stop and seek the advice of their doctor.

Proper Form and Alignment

Proper form and alignment are crucial for preventing injury and maximizing the benefits of exercise. When performing exercises, seniors should focus on keeping their spine in a neutral position, their shoulders relaxed, and their core engaged. They should also be mindful of their posture and avoid rounding their back or hunching forward.

It's also important for seniors to use the correct form when performing exercises. This can help reduce the risk of injury and ensure that they are getting the most benefit from their workout. If they are unsure of the correct form, they should seek the advice of a qualified instructor or physical therapist.

Avoiding Overuse Injuries and Common Exercise Pitfalls

When engaging in physical activity, it's important to be mindful of potential overuse injuries. This is especially true for seniors who may be more prone to these types of injuries due to age-related changes in the body. To minimize the risk of overuse injuries, it's important to gradually increase the intensity and duration of physical activity over time. This allows the body to adjust to the new demands placed on it, reducing the risk of injury.

Some common exercise pitfalls to be aware of include improper form, lack of proper stretching and warm-up exercises, and pushing yourself too hard too quickly. To avoid these pitfalls, it's important to seek guidance from a professional who can help you understand proper form and alignment and guide you in developing an appropriate exercise program.

Precautions for Seniors with Medical Conditions

Seniors with medical conditions, such as arthritis, heart disease, or respiratory problems, need to take special precautions when engaging in physical activity. In some cases, certain types of exercise may not be appropriate and alternative forms of exercise may need to be sought. For example, seniors with joint pain may find that low-impact activities, such as swimming or yoga, are more suitable for them than high-impact activities like running.

It's also important for seniors with medical conditions to consult with their healthcare provider before starting a new exercise program. This allows for a comprehensive assessment of the individual's health and fitness, as well as any special precautions or modifications that may be necessary.

<u>The Importance of Professional Guidance:</u>

Professional guidance is essential when it comes to developing a safe and effective exercise program for seniors. A professional can help seniors identify their fitness goals, design an appropriate exercise program, and ensure that the program is being executed safely and effectively.

In addition, a professional can provide ongoing support and guidance, helping seniors to stay motivated and on track with their exercise program. This can be especially helpful for seniors who may be new to exercise or who may have been inactive for a period of time.

Chapter 4

Pilates Routines

Seated Pilates Exercises

Pilates is a low-impact form of exercise that is perfect for seniors, especially those who have difficulty standing or have mobility issues. One of the ways that Pilates can be adapted for seniors is by performing the exercises while seated. Seated Pilates exercises are a great option for seniors who have difficulty standing, have mobility issues, or are recovering from an injury. In this sub-chapter, we'll discuss some of the most effective seated Pilates exercises and how they can benefit seniors over 60.

- **Seated Spine Twist**

The seated spine twist is a great exercise for seniors because it helps to increase flexibility and mobility in the spine. To perform this exercise, start by sitting in a chair with your feet flat on the ground and your hands resting on your knees. Next, twist your torso to one side, using your hands to gently push against your knee to deepen the stretch. Hold for a few seconds, and then release. Repeat on the other side. This exercise can be performed several times a day to improve spinal mobility and reduce the risk of falls.

- **Seated Arm Raise**

The seated arm raise is a simple exercise that can help to improve posture and increase upper body strength. To perform this exercise, start by sitting in a chair with your feet flat on the ground. Next, raise your arms straight up in front of you, reaching towards the ceiling. Hold for a few seconds, and then release. Repeat several times. This exercise can help to strengthen the muscles in your shoulders, arms, and upper back, which can help to reduce the risk of falls and improve your overall posture.

- **Seated Leg Raise**

The seated leg raise is another simple exercise that can help to improve strength and flexibility in the legs. To perform this exercise, start by sitting in a chair with your feet flat on the ground. Next, lift one leg straight up off the ground, holding for a few seconds. Release, and then repeat with the other leg. This exercise can help to strengthen the muscles in your legs, which can improve mobility and reduce the risk of falls.

- **Seated Hip Roll**

The seated hip roll is an exercise that can help to increase mobility in the hips and reduce the risk of falls. To perform this exercise, start by sitting in a chair with your feet flat on the ground. Next, roll your hips in a circular motion, using your hands to gently push against your knees for resistance. This exercise can help to improve hip mobility and reduce stiffness, which can reduce the risk of falls and improve overall mobility.

- **Cat and Cow Stretch**

Sit with your spine straight and your feet flat on the floor. Place your hands on your knees. On an inhale, drop your belly and lift your chin towards the ceiling, creating a "cow" shape. On an exhale, round your spine, tucking your chin towards your chest and making a "cat" shape. Repeat 5-10 times.

- **Neck Release**

Sit with your spine straight and your hands in your lap. Gently drop your right ear towards your right shoulder, holding the stretch for 5-10 seconds. Repeat on the left side.

- **Shoulder Roll**

Sit with your spine straight and your hands in your lap. Gently roll your shoulders forwards and backwards, then in a circle. Repeat 5-10 times.

- **Leg Lifts**

Sit with your spine straight and your feet flat on the floor. Lift one leg, holding it straight and keeping your foot flexed. Lower and repeat on the other leg.

- **Arm Lifts**

Sit with your spine straight and your hands resting on your knees. Lift one arm straight out in front of you, keeping it straight and parallel to the ground. Lower and repeat on the other arm.

These seated Pilates exercises are low-impact, making them ideal for seniors who may have difficulty with standing exercises. They can be performed anywhere with a chair and can help improve posture, flexibility, and balance.

Standing Pilates Exercises

Standing Pilates exercises are a great way to improve your balance and stability, as well as build strength and flexibility in the legs and core. These exercises are performed while standing, usually with the aid of a chair or wall for support. They can be easily adapted to accommodate different levels of ability, making them an ideal choice for seniors who are new to Pilates.

Some popular standing Pilates exercises include:

- **Wall-Supported Squats**

Stand facing a wall, with your feet hip-width apart and about a foot away from the wall. Slowly bend your knees and lower your body down as if you're sitting back into a chair. Push back up to the starting position, using your leg muscles to lift yourself. Repeat for 10-15 repetitions.

- **Wall-Supported Lunges**

Stand facing a wall, with one foot in front of the other. Bend the front knee, lowering your back knee toward the floor. Push back up to the starting position, and repeat with the other leg.

- **Wall-Supported Balancing**

Stand facing a wall, with one foot in front of the other. Raise your arms overhead and balance on one foot for 10-15 seconds, then switch to the other foot. Repeat for several repetitions.

- **Shoulder Blade Squeeze**

Stand with your feet hip-width apart, with your arms by your sides. Lift your shoulders up towards your ears, then squeeze your shoulder blades together and release. Repeat for 10-15 repetitions.

- **Standing Leg Raise**

Stand with your feet hip-width apart, and raise one leg straight out in front of you. Hold for a few seconds, then lower your leg and repeat with the other leg.

Incorporating these standing Pilates exercises into your routine can help improve your balance and stability, as well as strengthen the legs and core muscles. By using a wall or chair for support, you can safely and effectively perform these exercises, even if you have limited mobility or are recovering from an injury.

It is always important to consult with your doctor before starting any new exercise program, especially if you have any medical conditions or limitations. Additionally, working with a certified Pilates instructor can help ensure that you are performing the exercises safely and effectively, and can help you customize a routine that is specifically designed for your needs and abilities.

Mat-Based Pilates Exercises

Pilates mat work is a set of exercises that can be performed on a mat or floor. These exercises are designed to help improve balance, flexibility, and strength, and are often used to target specific areas of the body. Mat-based Pilates exercises are some of the most popular forms of Pilates and are perfect for seniors who are looking to get started with Pilates.

One of the benefits of mat-based Pilates exercises is that they can be easily modified to accommodate seniors with varying levels of fitness. For example, modifications can be made to make the exercises easier for seniors who are just starting out, or more challenging for those who are more advanced. In addition, mat-based Pilates exercises can be performed anywhere, making them an ideal choice for seniors who are looking for a convenient way to get started with Pilates.

Some of the most popular mat-based Pilates exercises include:

- **The Hundred**

This exercise is designed to improve core strength and stability. To perform the Hundred, start by lying on your back with your knees bent and your feet flat on the mat. Lift your head and shoulders off the mat, and then reach your arms up toward the ceiling. Perform 100 small, pulsing movements with your arms, making sure to keep your core engaged throughout the exercise.

- **The Roll-Up**

This exercise is designed to improve flexibility and balance. To perform the Roll-Up, start by lying on your back with your arms reaching up toward the ceiling. Reach forward to touch your toes, and then use your abs to roll up to a seated position. Repeat the exercise several times, making sure to keep your movements slow and controlled.

- **The Single-Leg Circle**

This exercise is designed to improve balance and stability. To perform the Single-Leg Circle, start by lying on your back with your legs extended. Lift one leg off the mat, and then use your abs to circle the leg in a controlled manner. Repeat the exercise several times on each leg.

- **The Double-Leg Stretch**

This exercise is designed to improve flexibility and balance. To perform the Double-Leg Stretch, start by lying on your back with your legs extended. Reach your arms forward, and then use your abs to lift your legs off the mat. Reach your legs toward the ceiling, and then use your abs to reach them back toward the mat. Repeat the exercise several times, making sure to keep your movements slow and controlled.

Pilates Workouts for Different Levels of Ability

Pilates can be a highly adaptable form of exercise, making it suitable for seniors of all fitness levels. Whether you are a beginner, have an injury, or are looking for a challenging workout, there is a Pilates routine that can be tailored to meet your needs. Here are some examples of Pilates workouts designed for different levels of ability:

- **Beginner Pilates Workout**

For those who are new to Pilates, it is important to start with a beginner-friendly routine. This workout should focus on basic movements that can help you build strength, flexibility, and balance. Some examples of beginner Pilates exercises include the knee roll, the spine stretch, and the pelvic tilt.

- **Pilates Workout for Injury Recovery**

If you have a recent injury or chronic pain, it is important to choose exercises that are safe and gentle. Pilates can be a great choice for injury recovery because it can help you build strength and flexibility without putting too much stress on your injured area. Some examples of Pilates exercises for injury recovery include the pelvic tilt, the cat stretch, and the standing hip flexor stretch.

- **Intermediate Pilates Workout**

Once you have built up some strength and confidence, you may be ready to move on to an intermediate Pilates workout. This workout should focus on more challenging movements that can help you build endurance and stability. Some examples of intermediate Pilates exercises include the single leg stretch, the double leg stretch, and the swan dive.

- **Advanced Pilates Workout**

For those who are looking for a challenge, an advanced Pilates workout may be just what you need. This workout should include complex movements that require a high level of strength, flexibility, and coordination. Some examples of advanced Pilates exercises include the roll-up, the teaser, and the mermaid.

Regardless of your fitness level, it is important to listen to your body and choose exercises that feel safe and comfortable. If you have any medical conditions or injuries, it is also important to seek the advice of a professional Pilates instructor before starting any new workout routine.

Creating a Custom Pilates Routine

Creating a custom Pilates routine is a great way to make Pilates exercise more personalized and tailored to your specific needs and goals. Whether you are a beginner or an experienced Pilates practitioner, a custom routine can help you achieve your desired outcomes more effectively and efficiently. There are several key steps to creating a custom Pilates routine, which include:

- **Assess Your Fitness Level:**

Before you start creating your Pilates routine, it's important to assess your current fitness level. This will help you determine the types of exercises and workouts that are appropriate for you and your needs. You should take into account your physical capabilities, any medical conditions, and any injuries or other limitations you may have.

- **Determine Your Goals:**

What do you want to achieve through Pilates exercise? Do you want to improve your flexibility, strength, balance, or posture? Do you have a specific health condition you're trying to manage? Having a clear understanding of your goals will help you create a routine that is tailored to your needs and will help you achieve the outcomes you're looking for.

- **Choose the Right Pilates Equipment:**

Pilates can be done with or without equipment. If you choose to use equipment, such as a Pilates reformer, it's important to select the right equipment for your fitness level and goals. You should also consider the cost, storage, and ease of use of each piece of equipment.

- **Choose the Right Exercises:**

Once you have assessed your fitness level and determined your goals, you can begin selecting the right Pilates exercises for your routine. You should choose exercises that are appropriate for your fitness level and that will help you achieve your desired outcomes. You can also consult a Pilates instructor or a Pilates reference book for guidance on selecting the right exercises.

- **Plan Your Routine:**

Once you have chosen your Pilates exercises, you can start putting together your routine. You should aim to create a routine that is well-rounded and that includes exercises that work on your flexibility, strength, balance, and posture. You should also consider the intensity and duration of your workouts, as well as any modifications you may need to make to accommodate your fitness level and any limitations you may have.

- **Incorporate Variety:**

To prevent boredom and help you stay motivated, it's important to incorporate a variety of exercises and workouts into your Pilates routine. You can switch up your routine by changing the order of your exercises, adding new exercises, or trying new equipment. You can also try different types of Pilates, such as mat-based, reformer-based, or chair-based Pilates.

- **Get Professional Guidance:**

Pilates is a safe and effective form of exercise, but it's important to get professional guidance from a Pilates instructor to ensure that you are doing the exercises correctly and safely. A Pilates instructor can also help you create a custom Pilates routine that is tailored to your needs and goals, and can provide ongoing support and guidance to help you achieve the best possible outcomes.

By following these steps, you can create a custom Pilates routine that is tailored to your needs and that will help you achieve your desired outcomes. Whether you're a beginner or an experienced Pilates practitioner, a custom routine is an effective way to make Pilates exercise more personal and rewarding.

Incorporating Pilates into Your Daily Routine

One of the best things about Pilates is that it can be easily integrated into your daily routine, regardless of your lifestyle or schedule. Whether you are a busy professional or a retiree, you can find ways to make Pilates a part of your daily life. Here are some tips to help you get started:

- **Start slow:**

Don't try to do too much too soon. Start with a few simple exercises and gradually work your way up to more complex routines.

- **Make it a habit:**

Set aside a specific time each day for Pilates and stick to it. This will help you establish a routine and make it easier to stick with.

- **Use a Pilates DVD or online video:**

There are many excellent Pilates videos available online or on DVD that can guide you through various routines. These can be a great way to get started and to stay motivated.

- **Join a class:**

Consider joining a Pilates class, especially if you are a beginner. This will give you the opportunity to learn from an experienced instructor and to interact with other Pilates enthusiasts.

- **Practice at home:**

You can easily practice Pilates at home using a mat or other props. This can be a convenient way to get in some exercise when you are short on time or when it's not feasible to go to a class.

- **Mix it up:**

To avoid boredom and to challenge your body in different ways, try incorporating a variety of Pilates exercises into your routine. This can help you target different muscle groups and improve your overall fitness level.

- **Get professional guidance:**

Consider working with a Pilates instructor to help you create a customized routine that is tailored to your specific needs and goals. This can be especially beneficial if you have any medical conditions or injuries.

Incorporating Pilates into your daily routine can be a fun and effective way to stay active and improve your overall health and well-being. With a little bit of effort and discipline, you can enjoy the many benefits of Pilates for years to come.

Chapter 5
Staying Motivated

Setting Realistic Goals

Staying motivated is an important part of any fitness program, especially for seniors who are just starting out with Pilates. One of the best ways to keep your motivation levels high is to set realistic goals for yourself. By setting achievable targets, you will be more likely to stick to your Pilates routine and see progress over time.

When setting your goals, it's important to consider your current fitness level, any physical limitations, and your overall health. For example, if you have limited mobility, you may want to focus on seated Pilates exercises or mat-based exercises that can be modified to accommodate your needs. On the other hand, if you are relatively fit, you may want to aim for standing Pilates exercises or more advanced Pilates workouts.

It's also important to set realistic time frames for your goals. For example, you may not be able to complete a full Pilates routine on your first day, but with time and practice, you can work towards longer and more challenging workouts. Similarly, if you have a physical limitation, it may take you longer to see results than someone who does not have the same issue.

Another way to stay motivated is to track your progress. Keep a journal of your workouts and take note of any improvements you see over time. This could be anything from increased flexibility, improved balance, or even better posture. By keeping track of your progress, you will be able to see just how far you have come, and this can be a great source of motivation.

Finally, it's important to find a workout buddy or join a Pilates class. Having someone to exercise with can make your Pilates routine more fun and enjoyable, and it can also help to keep you accountable. If you can't find someone to workout with, consider joining a Pilates class. This will give you the opportunity to meet new people and learn from a professional instructor.

Finding a Workout Buddy

Finding a workout buddy can be a great way to stay motivated and make exercising a more enjoyable experience. When you have a partner to exercise with, it provides accountability and encourages you to stick to your routine. This can help you push through tough workouts, stay committed to your exercise plan, and ultimately achieve your fitness goals.

Having a workout buddy can also make exercise more fun and engaging. You can motivate each other, share your progress, and help each other stay motivated. Furthermore, you can try new exercises together and help each other with proper form and technique. This can not only make your workouts more effective but also help prevent injury.

When selecting a workout buddy, it's important to choose someone who is supportive, encouraging, and has similar fitness goals. You want to work with someone who is just as dedicated to their own fitness as you are, and who will help you stay accountable. It's also helpful to find someone who you enjoy spending time with, as this will make your workouts much more enjoyable.

It's important to keep in mind that not everyone is a good fit as a workout buddy. Some people may not be as dedicated or may not have the same level of fitness. If your workout buddy becomes more of a hindrance than a help, it's okay to end the partnership and find someone new. The goal is to find someone who motivates and encourages you, not someone who causes you stress or frustration.

Tracking Progress

One of the key factors in staying motivated is to track progress. This helps you see the improvements you've made over time and keeps you focused on your goals.

When it comes to Pilates, tracking progress can be done in several ways, including:

- **Keeping a journal:**

Keeping a journal of your Pilates routines and noting any changes in your abilities and flexibility can be a great way to track progress. This can be as simple as writing down the exercises you did, how many repetitions, and any modifications you made.

- **Taking measurements:**

Another way to track progress is by taking regular measurements of your body, such as your waist size, hip size, and thigh size. By measuring these areas, you can see if your Pilates routine is helping you achieve your desired results.

- **Taking photos:**

Taking regular photos can also be a great way to track progress. This is especially useful for tracking changes in your posture and body shape. You can take photos before you start your Pilates routine, and then every few weeks or months to see the changes.

- **Monitoring strength and flexibility:**

Another way to track progress is by monitoring your strength and flexibility. You can do this by checking how many repetitions of an exercise you can do, or how long you can hold a stretch. This can give you a good indication of whether your Pilates routine is helping you improve in these areas.

- **Working with a professional:**

A Pilates instructor can help you track your progress by providing feedback on your form and technique. They can also provide you with customized routines to help you reach your goals more effectively.

By tracking your progress, you can stay motivated and focused on your Pilates goals. Whether you choose to keep a journal, take measurements, take photos, monitor your strength and flexibility, or work with a professional, tracking progress is a key component to success in your Pilates journey.

Celebrating Success

One of the most important aspects of staying motivated in any fitness or wellness journey is to celebrate your successes along the way. When you set realistic goals for yourself and work hard to achieve them, it is important to take time to acknowledge and celebrate your progress. This not only reinforces the positive changes you are making in your life, but it also provides motivation to continue your journey.

Incorporating Pilates into your daily routine can bring a sense of accomplishment and satisfaction, especially as you begin to see improvements in your posture, mobility, and overall physical and mental well-being. Celebrating your successes along the way can help keep you motivated and on track.

Here are some tips to help you celebrate your Pilates successes:

- **Take note of your progress:**

Keep a journal or record of your Pilates routine, including the exercises you do, the number of repetitions, and how you feel before and after each session. As you progress, look back at your journal and see how far you have come.

- **Share your progress with friends and family:**

Share your Pilates journey with loved ones who will support and encourage you. Share your progress and talk about how Pilates has positively impacted your life.

- **Reward yourself:**

Treat yourself to something special when you reach a milestone, such as a new outfit to wear to Pilates class, a relaxing massage, or a special treat.

- **Celebrate with a Pilates class or workout:**

Dedicate a Pilates session to celebrate your progress and to focus on your goals. Use the class or workout as a way to reflect on your journey and to look forward to the future.

Celebrating your successes in Pilates can help keep you motivated and on track, so be sure to take the time to acknowledge your progress and celebrate your accomplishments. Whether it is with friends, family, or simply by yourself, make sure you celebrate your successes and enjoy the journey.

Overcoming Plateaus and Setbacks

When it comes to any exercise routine, including Pilates, it is common for people to reach a plateau in their progress. This can be a discouraging experience, but it is important to remember that it is a normal part of the process. Plateaus can occur when the body has become too familiar with the exercises being performed, causing the progress to slow down. To overcome this, it is important to change up the routine by adding new exercises or increasing the difficulty of the current exercises. This will challenge the body in new ways, resulting in continued progress.

Another common setback in any exercise routine is injury. This can be caused by overuse or poor form during exercises. To prevent injury, it is important to listen to the body and never push through pain. It is also important to be aware of proper form and alignment during exercises to reduce the risk of injury. If an injury does occur, it is best to seek guidance from a professional and take the necessary time to properly recover before returning to exercise.

Staying Committed to Pilates

Staying committed to a Pilates routine can be a challenge, especially for seniors who may have other responsibilities and commitments. However, the benefits of Pilates make it worth sticking with the routine. To stay committed, it is helpful to set achievable goals and track progress. Having a workout buddy can also provide accountability and motivation to stick with the routine. It is also important to celebrate successes and acknowledge the progress made.

Incorporating Pilates into daily life can help make the routine more sustainable and enjoyable. This can be as simple as incorporating small Pilates exercises into daily activities, such as stretching before getting out of bed in the morning or doing a few balancing exercises throughout the day. Staying committed to Pilates can also be made easier by finding a workout environment that is enjoyable and supportive, such as a Pilates class or a workout group.

It is important to remember that the benefits of Pilates take time and consistent effort. However, by staying committed and making it a part of daily life, the results can be significant and long-lasting. Improving physical health, reducing the risk of falls and age-related conditions, and improving overall quality of life are just a few of the benefits that can be gained from staying committed to a Pilates routine.

Chapter 6

Pilates Equipment and Props

Understanding the Different Pilates Props

Pilates equipment and props are an important aspect of a Pilates workout. There are various types of props available in the market that can enhance the effectiveness of your Pilates practice and make it easier to perform certain exercises. Some of the most commonly used Pilates props include Pilates balls, resistance bands, Pilates rings, foam rollers, and stability balls.

Each prop has a different purpose and is designed to target specific muscle groups and movements. Pilates balls, for instance, are often used to target the deep muscles in your core, hips, and back. Resistance bands can help you increase resistance during exercises, making your workout more challenging. Pilates rings are used to increase resistance on specific areas, such as your arms and legs, while foam rollers help to release tension in your muscles and increase flexibility.

It is important to understand the different Pilates props and how they can be used to get the most out of your workout. Before you start using Pilates props, make sure to familiarize yourself with proper usage, as improper use can lead to injury.

Choosing the Right Pilates Equipment for Your Needs

When choosing Pilates equipment, it is important to consider your fitness level, any medical conditions you may have, and your individual goals. For example, if you have lower back pain, a foam roller or stability ball may be a better choice than a Pilates ring.

It is also important to consider the cost of the equipment and whether it is a good investment for your Pilates practice. While some props, like Pilates balls and resistance bands, are relatively inexpensive, others, like Pilates reformers, can be quite costly.

It is always a good idea to speak with a professional Pilates instructor before making a purchase, as they can provide guidance on which props will best suit your needs. Additionally, they can demonstrate proper usage and help you integrate the props into your Pilates routine.

Ultimately, the right Pilates equipment and props can enhance your Pilates practice, making it more effective and enjoyable. With the right props and equipment, you can effectively target specific muscle groups, increase resistance, and improve your overall fitness level.

Making the Most of Your Pilates Props

Pilates equipment and props can greatly enhance your workout and help you achieve your fitness goals. However, it is important to understand how to make the most of these props and use them correctly. In this section, we will explore the various Pilates props and how they can be used to achieve maximum benefits.

Pilates props include items such as resistance bands, Pilates balls, foam rollers, Pilates rings, and more. Each of these props can be used in a variety of exercises to increase resistance, provide support, or add a challenge to your workout.

- **Resistance Bands:**

Resistance bands are versatile props that can be used to add resistance to your Pilates workouts. They come in different levels of resistance and can be used for a variety of exercises, including arm and leg movements, as well as core strengthening exercises. When using resistance bands, it is important to choose the right level of resistance for your fitness level and to make sure you are using proper form to avoid injury.

- **Pilates Balls:**

Pilates balls are small, inflatable balls that can be used to add an extra challenge to your workout. They can be used for balance exercises, core strengthening exercises, and more. When using Pilates balls, it is important to start with a smaller ball and gradually work your way up to a larger ball as your strength and stability improve.

- **Foam Rollers:**

Foam rollers are long, cylindrical props that can be used for massage and self-myofascial release. They can be used to massage and stretch tight muscles, relieve tension, and improve flexibility. When using foam rollers, it is important to start with a softer foam roller and gradually work your way up to a firmer foam roller as your strength and flexibility improve.

- **Pilates Rings:**

Pilates rings are circular props that can be used for a variety of exercises, including arm and leg movements, as well as core strengthening exercises. Pilates rings provide resistance and can help to improve your posture, balance, and stability. When using Pilates rings, it is important to start with a lighter resistance and gradually work your way up to a heavier resistance as your strength and stability improve.

Incorporating Pilates props into your workout can be a great way to increase the intensity and challenge of your Pilates routine. However, it is important to use proper form and to start with a lighter resistance before gradually increasing the intensity. With the right Pilates props and the right approach, you can achieve your fitness goals and take your Pilates workout to the next level.

Conclusion

In conclusion, Pilates is a low-impact form of exercise that can provide numerous benefits to seniors. It is an effective way to improve flexibility, balance, strength, and overall health. The exercises can be modified to accommodate different levels of ability and can be performed with or without equipment. Pilates routines can be customized to meet individual goals and preferences, making it an enjoyable form of exercise. Staying motivated is an important part of any exercise program, and Pilates is no exception. Setting realistic goals, finding a workout buddy, tracking progress, and celebrating success can help seniors stay committed to their Pilates practice. It is also important to understand the different Pilates props and choose the right equipment for your needs. With the help of professional guidance, Pilates can be an excellent way for seniors to maintain their physical and mental health. This book has provided an overview of the many benefits of Pilates and how it can be incorporated into a daily routine for maximum benefits. Whether you are a beginner or have been practicing Pilates for some time, this book has provided you with valuable information and resources to help you reach your goals.

www.ingramcontent.com/pod-product-compliance
Lightning Source LLC
Chambersburg PA
CBHW071550260726

48653CB00007BA/2713